1

2

How to make 11 favorite salad recipes

COPYRIGHT NOTICE

TABLE OF CONTENTS

CURTIDO

A curtido is a simple salad served with plain bread. The restaurant keeps a large jar of curtido and serves a variety of dishes in addition to salad. Curtido is usually lightly fermented at room temperature before serving, resulting in a type of Salvadoran cabbage.

Ingredients

Finely chopped cabbage - 1/2 cup

Peeled and chopped carrots - 1

Boiled water - 4 cups

Finely chopped green onion - 3

White vinegar - 1/2 cup

Water - 1/2 cup

Finely chopped jalapeño or serrano peppers - 1

Salt - 1/2 tsp

Method

1. Place the cabbage and carrots in a large heatproof bowl. Pour enough boiling water into a bowl to cover the cabbage and carrots and leave for about 5 minutes. Place in a colander and squeeze out as much water as possible.

2. Return the cabbage and carrots to the bowl and toss with the remaining ingredients. If desired, leave at room temperature for several hours or overnight. Let it cool down and serve as a pupusa side dish.

CAUSA RELLENA

This versatile Peruvian potato dish is a delicious side dish or a great addition to a buffet. Causa can be layered with any number of fillings. Chicken salad and tuna salad are popular menu items. When served cold, the dish is often topped with colorful garnishes and sauces to give it a colorful flavor.

Ingredients

Yellow potatoes (Yukon Gold) - 2 pounds

Oil - 1/2 cup

Lemon or lime juice - 1/4 cup

Salt and pepper to taste

Boiled eggs, cut into rounds - 2 to 3

Ground black olives - 6 to 8

Method

1. Place the potatoes in a large pot of cold, salted water. Bring to the boil and cook until the potatoes are soft and tender. Drain and cool.

2. Once the potatoes are cool enough to handle, you can peel them. Mash the potatoes using a masher or potato masher until smooth. Mix the oil, red pepper paste, lemon or lime juice, salt and pepper to taste.

3. Line a baking sheet or tray with plastic wrap and press to fit in the dish. Place half of the potatoes on the bottom of the plate and flatten them. Spread desired filling evenly over potatoes. Spread the remaining potatoes evenly over the filling. Press gently to see why. Cover and cool completely.

4. Place a serving plate upside down on top of the causa dish. Using both hands, turn the bowl upside down and lower the bowl into the bowl. Remove and discard the plastic wrap.

5. Garnish the cause with boiled eggs and olives and add sauce if desired. Cut into pieces and serve.

POTATO SALAD

Potato salad is the American picnic and barbecue favorite. The basic recipe for fried potatoes thickened with mayonnaise and served cold is also found in northern Germany. There are many different potato salad recipes, but here are some basic recipes you can put together.

Ingredients

Boil, peel and cut the potatoes into large pieces - 2 kilograms.

Thinly sliced red onion - 1/2

Mayonnaise - 1 cup

Red or white vinegar - 2 tablespoons

Salt - 1 1/2 tsp

Pepper - 1/2 tsp

Method

1. Place the potatoes in a large saucepan and cover with cold water. Add a large pinch of salt and bring to a boil over medium-high heat. Once the water is boiling, reduce the heat to low and simmer until cooked through and tender, about 10 to 20 minutes. Once a sharp knife slides easily in and out of a test piece of potato, it's ready. Drain the potatoes in a colander and let them steam dry for about 5 minutes.

2. Combine potatoes and remaining ingredients in a large bowl and toss together. Mash the potatoes a bit, but leave most of them in chunks.

3. Adjust seasoning to taste, then chill and enjoy.

SWEET COLESLAW

Sweet coleslaw is a type of salad that is different from other salads that do not contain mayonnaise.

Ingredients

Chopped onion - 1/2

Sugar - 1/2 cup

Dry mustard - 2 tsp

Celery seeds - 1-2 teaspoons

Salt, pepper - for seasoning

Cider vinegar - 1/2 cup

Oil - 1/2 cup

Finely chopped cabbage - 1 head

Peeled and chopped carrots - 2-3

Method

1. Place the onion, sugar, mustard, celery seed, salt and pepper in a blender. While the blender is running, slowly pour the oil through the top hole. Adjust the seasoning of the emulsified sauce.

2. Place the shredded cabbage and carrots in a large bowl and toss with the dressing. Cover and let cool completely before serving.

BEEF SALPICON

Popular in Central America, salpicon is a refreshing salad that is delicious as a topping on tostadas or wrapped in fresh corn tortillas. It is very easy to make in bulk for parties or

18

family gatherings.

Ingredients

Beef or skirt steak - 2-2 1/2 lbs

Chopped onion - 1

Olive oil - 1/3 cup

Vinegar - 1/4 cup

Oregano - 1-2 teaspoons

Salt and pepper to taste

Tomatoes cut without seeds - 3

Thinly sliced onion - 1

Serrano pepper, crushed or mashed - 3

Finely chopped avocado - 2

Method

1. Place the beef, onion and salt in a large pot and add enough water to cover. Bring to a boil, then reduce the heat to medium and simmer for 1 1/2 to 2 hours or until the meat is very tender. Remove the meat and reserve the broth for soup or other recipes. Once cool enough to handle, crush the meat with your fingers.

2. In a large bowl, whisk together the olive oil, vinegar, oregano, salt, and pepper. Add the tomatoes, chopped onion and hot pepper and mix. Let the vegetables marinate for a few minutes.

3. Gently toss the beef and avocado with the pickled vegetables and seasonings. Spread on a baking tray and serve cold or warm with scones at room temperature.

TABOULI

A light, refreshing and healthy Middle Eastern salad, tabouli is made with bulgur, chopped parsley and peas, tossed with lemon juice and olive oil.

Ingredients

Bulgur - 3/4 cup

Hot water - 3 cups

Finely chopped flat-leaf parsley – 3 bunches

Tomatoes cut without seeds - 2

Chopped green onions - 4 to 6

Lemon juice - 1/2 cup

Salt and pepper to taste

Olive oil - 1/2 cup

Method

1. Place the bulgur in a large bowl and cover with water. Let it stand for 20-30 minutes and then drain. Place the soaked cauliflower in a clean cloth and wring out the moisture. Return the bulgur to the bowl.

2. Add the parsley, tomatoes, green onion, lemon juice, salt and pepper and mix. Let sit for 15-20 minutes until flavors meld.

3. Adjust seasoning and add olive oil. Serve cold or at room temperature.

White Bean & Tuna Salad with Basil Vinaigrette

Ingredients

Kosher salt and pepper

12 ounces green beans, trimmed and halved

1 small shallot, chopped

1 o'clock Lightly dried basil leaves

3 spoons. olive oil

1 spoon. red wine vinegar

Torn salad at 16:00

1 15 ounces small white kidney beans, rinsed

2 5-ounce cans of albacore tuna in water

4 soft-boiled eggs, cut in half

Method

1. Bring a large pot of water to a boil. Add 1 tablespoon salt, add green beans, and cook until tender, 3 to 4 minutes. Drain, rinse in cold water and cool.

2. Meanwhile, puree shallots, basil, oil, vinegar, 1/2 teaspoon salt, and pepper in a blender until smooth.

3. Place half of the mixture in a large bowl and toss with the green beans. Toss the lettuce,

white beans and tuna and serve with the remaining dressing and the eggs.

Vegan Ceaser Salad

This is a fun dinner that everyone can enjoy, regardless of their dietary preferences (meat lovers will love this too!).

Ingredients

For crispy chickpeas

1 15-ounce can of beans

1 spoon olive oil

Kosher salt and pepper

1/2 tsp grated lemon peel before getting dressed

For dressing

1/4 p. olive oil

1 teaspoon Grated lemon peel and 1/3 cup

lemon juice

1/4 tsp tahini

1 spoon nutritional yeast

1 spoon Dijon mustard

2 teaspoons caper 1 teaspoon of caper brine

1 teaspoon of finely chopped garlic

Kosher salt and pepper

For the salad

4 slices of thick bread

3 spoons olive oil

2 small red onions, thickly sliced

Kosher salt and pepper

2 bundles of small radishes

1 clove of garlic, half

2 hearts of green or romaine lettuce, the leaves separated

Method

Make crispy chickpeas:

1. Preheat oven to 425° F. Rinse the chickpeas. Pat dry with paper towels and discard any loose skin.

2. On a rimmed baking sheet, toss the chickpeas with the olive oil and 1/4 teaspoon salt and pepper. Bake, stirring occasionally, until crisp, 30 to 40 minutes.

3. Remove from the oven, put in a bowl and mix with lemon peel. Chickpeas remain crunchy even when cooled.

Prepare the dressing and salad:

1. Heat grill to medium-high. Make the

dressing: Place all dressing ingredients in a small blender or food processor and puree until smooth, then add water 1 tablespoon at a time to adjust consistency and season with salt and pepper. Keep dressing separate.

2. To make the salad: Brush the bread with 1 1/2 teaspoons oil. Brush the onion slices with 1 tablespoon oil and season with 1/4 teaspoon salt and pepper. Season the radishes with the remaining 1/2 tablespoon of oil and a pinch of salt. Cut the radishes into small skewers. Cook the bread until browned, 2 to 3 minutes per side. Rub immediately with garlic. Cook the onion and radish until soft. Fry the onions for about 5 minutes on each side and the radishes for about 6 to 8 minutes on each side.

3. Slice the bread and release the onion rings. Add half of the dressing to the lettuce and

toss. Carefully fold in the toasted croutons and onion rings. Serve with radish skewers, crispy chickpeas and remaining sauce for drizzling or dipping.

Winter Green Salad

This fresh and flavorful salad goes well with

big meat dishes and is loaded with hearty vegetables like frisée, endive, and radicchio. Chopped sweet pecans, aged gouda and a simple vinaigrette complete this salad for a satisfying finish.

Ingredients:

3 spoons sherry vinegar

2 teaspoons Rustic Dijon mustard

1 1/2 teaspoon honey

Kosher salt and pepper

1/4 p olive oil1 small red onion, thinly sliced

1 small french fry (about 3 ounces), trimmed and cut into small pieces

1 head of Boston or Little Gem lettuce (about 200g), leaves trimmed and torn

2 heads of red endive, trimmed and leaves separated

1 cup (about 6 ounces) Castelfranco radicchio, chopped, leaves torn

1/2 p Candied pecans, coarsely chopped

2 ounces shaved old gouda

Method

1. In a medium bowl, whisk together the vinegar, mustard, honey, 3/4 teaspoon salt, and 1/2 teaspoon pepper. Slowly pour in the oil and beat until smooth. Add the onion and leave for 15 minutes

2. Meanwhile, in a very large bowl (or dividing into two large bowls if necessary) toss the

frisée, lettuce, endives and radicchio until well combined. Add dressing and toss to combine. Serve with pecans and gouda.

COBB SALAD

Cobb salad is an American garden salad typically made with chopped lettuce, tomato, bacon, chicken breast, hard-boiled egg, avocado, onion, blue cheese, and red wine vinaigrette. The ingredients are arranged on the plate. Served as a main course.

Ingredients

6 bacon slices

3 eggs

1 head of iceberg lettuce, chopped

3 cups of chopped boiled chicken

2 tomatoes, seeded and chopped

¼ cup shredded blue cheese

3 chopped green onions

1 avocado - peeled, mashed and diced

1 bottle (8 ounces) Ranch-style salad dressing

Method

1. Put eggs in a saucepan and cover completely with cold water. Bring to a boil, cover and remove from heat. Let the eggs stand for 10-12 minutes, then cool, then peel and finely chop.

2. While the eggs are cooking, place the bacon in a large, deep pan. Cook over medium heat until evenly browned, 7 to 10 minutes. Drain, chop and set aside.

3. Divide the chopped salad among individual plates. Top with bacon, eggs, chicken, tomatoes, blue cheese, green onions and avocado.

4. Drizzle with dressing.